# The Regimen for Good Health and Longevity

## ---Keep Doctors and Drugs Away

# Contents

**Preface**

**Chapter I    Cultivating Mentality**

**Chapter II    Proper Food Taking**

**Chapter III    Right Ways of Life**

**Chapter IV    Foot Bathing ---Soaking Feet**

Section 1    Introduction of Foot Bathing and Its Benefits

Section 2    TCM Prescriptions for Foot Bathing

Section 3    Scientific Basis for Foot Bathing Regimen

**Chapter V    Conclusion**



*Regimen of Good Health and Longevity*

# Preface

Good health and longevity are the aspirations of all people from the ancient times to the present.   Due to the low development level of science and technology, particularly the medical technology in ancient time, the life span of ancients is not long compared with the modern people. Since the industrial revolution, the world science and technology has been advancing with great leap. Today, the world has entered into the high-tech and information era. The high technologies promote the wealth growth with unprecedented rate and bring about the convenient and quick life to people. However, more and more people do not feel happy, quiet and peaceful in mind, high-technologies do not take health to people although medical technologies and means are becoming more and more advanced, people are still plagued by various unidentified diseases and virus that are coming up one after another, the number of patients is still rising. Many people could do nothing but wait for death when a serious disease befalls them. What are the underlying reasons for that?

Human life, in essence, is a most sophisticated and advanced movement on the Earth, so all men need to acquire the energy from the natural all the time, namely the food, drink and various necessities, for maintaining the life movement or survival, so, it is the fundamental interest of human for survival and safety. Besides, human has various desires to be satisfied all the time. In this connection, pursuit of interest and satisfaction of desires are the natural characters of human and constitute the engine of life. As all men are pursuing their interest and trying to satisfy their desires as much as possible, the competition and struggle between men for maximizing their interest and satisfaction of desires are inevitable. Under fierce social completion and great pressure for safety and survival, many people are racked with anxiety, causing the psychology and mental problems. Human health includes physical health and mental health and is closely associated with the food, psychology and mentality of human. The sickness of man today is more than a problem of human body working, it is a problem jointly caused by mental state, social operation, human relations, personal quality and other factors, it is, to some extent, is a social problem. The resistance and immunity are the self-protection mechanism of human body. To resist the disease and virus, the resistance and immunity of human body are essential. In order to enhance the resistance and immunity of human body, **Cultivating Mentality, Taking Proper Food, Following Right Ways of Life and Regular Foot Bathing** for such purposes are fundamental and crucial. The ultimate purposes of regimen are to make preventive treatment of future or possible diseases, or to prevent diseases, or to keep diseases away, and achieve good health and longevity without going to a doctor and taking medicines. Prevention excels treatment and regimen means longevity. So, the regimen is more than the skills of protecting human body for good health and longevity. It is a great way of life. So long as these ways of enhancing the resistance and immunity of human body are followed, the good health and longevity are no longer an objective beyond reach.



*Regimen of Good Health and Longevity*

# Chapter I   Cultivating Mentality

The facts and scientific research indicate that emotional disorder injures the internal organs of human body. Among the internal organs, the liver is the first one that feels and responds to the emotion changes. The slight or positive emotion changes produce no negative impact on the liver, but the negative emotion changes will injure the liver first, causing the dysfunction of Qi (vital energy) of the liver and detriment to the health of human body. It is similar to the situation that the climate will change when the atmosphere flow is blocked or is not smooth, leading to the outbreak of natural disasters and pandemics. To some extent, atmosphere is the Qi of the Earth. The dysfunction of Qi of the liver inhibits the smooth flow of spleen and stomach, causing the discomforts of human body, such as abdominal distention, hypochondriac pain, slight ache and lack of appetite, etc. The spleen and stomach are the foundation of acquired constitution and the source of qi and blood formation. When the spleen and stomach have problem, the immunity weakens, the human body is vulnerable to various diseases and viruses. So, keeping a good mood is primary to good health.

Sitting still as a form of therapy (meditation) is a good way of regulating the mentality or mood. It can pacify and soothe the emotion, enhance the "Defense Qi of Human Body" and strengthen the immunity.

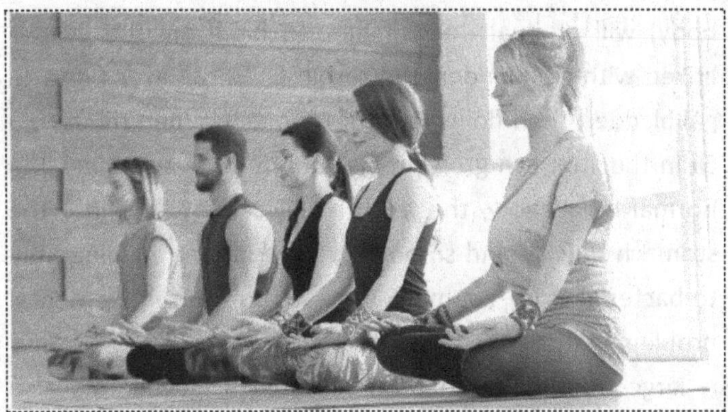

Sitting still as a form of therapy can pacify and soothe the emotion, enhance the "Defense Qi of Human Body" and strengthen the immunity

There are a few cases proving that many diseases are caused by mentality. Why someone gets gastric ulcer? The reason is that his stomach cannot receive the fresh blood smoothly and quickly. Fresh blood is the best repairing tool of human organs as it contains antibody, phagocyte that kills the pathogens, and nutrition, etc. What is the reason that the stomach cannot receive fresh blood? According to "Huang Di Canon of Internal Medicine (Huang Di Nei Jing)", the first classic work of Traditional Chinese Medicine and crowned as "Ancestor of Medicine' and "Cornerstone Work of Traditional Chinese Medicine, wrath hurts the liver. If someone gets angry and complains from time to time, the turbid Qi (According to the theory of Traditional Chinese Medicine, Qi, also known as Vital Energy, is a very nutritive refined substance that has strong vitality and moves endlessly throughout the whole human body, it is a basic constituent substance of human body and it maintains, promotes, stimulates and regulates the life activity of human body, it is the vital energy of human

5

body) will gradually accumulate in his liver. The liver is linked with gallbladder, the turbid Qi in the liver flows to gallbladder, then flows into the stomach. When the turbid Qi in the stomach grows more and more, it will block the normal blood flow, the fresh blood cannot flow into the stomach quickly and smoothly, the stomach is vulnerable to bacterial virus. So, many diseases are caused by mental problem in most circumstances.

A large number of medical research achievements also indicate that 80% of diseases are caused by mental factors, only 20% of the same are caused by outside factors, including bacterial infections.

Someone once did such experiment: hang up a monkey and give electric stimulation to it, getting the monkey in an anxious mood. Soon, the money got the gastric ulcer, then use the Gastrofiberscope, X-Ray, electroencephalogram and biochemistry to analyze the pathological mechanism, finding that the occurrence of gastric disease is closely associated with hyper-excitability or suppression of cerebral cortex, and vegetative nerve functional disturbance.

Just as described in the "Huang Di Canon of Internal Medicine (Huang Di Nei Jing)": wrath impairs the liver, over joy impairs the heart, over sorrow impairs the lungs, big fright and dread impair the kidney, excessive nostalgia impairs the spleen; wrath drives Qi flow upward (blood pressure rises), over joy makes Qi slack, grief consumes Qi, dread drives Qi flow downward (blood pressure falls), fright disorders Qi (it might lead to the breathing break, causing death) and over sorrow stagnates Qi (it might lead to the halt of Qi and flood flow, causing death), most of diseases are caused by mental problem, the mood and mind of human produce direct impact on the health status of human body. So, "Cultivating Mentality" is primary for improving the immunity, maintaining good health and achieving longevity, it is complementary with medical treatment in controlling and curing the diseases. To cultivate the mentality, one must do the things below:

**First, Refrain from Discomposure.** When the discomposure comes up, the human organs will become abnormal. The peaceful mind generates harmonious Qi, harmonious Qi promotes smooth blood flow, the smooth blood flow brings about sufficient vital essence and sufficient vital essence produces vigorous spirit, namely "Being Energetic". Only in such mental state, the resistance and immunity of human body are very strong to the diseases and viruses, that is, the vital essence is strong. So long as one can remain a peaceful mind and keep calm and confident    when a disease or a trouble befalls him, it will no longer be a problem for him. Those who understand the life wisdom and way of life usually have better health and longer life span, the reason for which is that they know the operating logic of the world and all things and realize that misfortune is a part of life, ups and downs are the normal state of life. So, they can remain a peaceful mind and keep calm in face of misfortune.

All things have their respective laws and experience the stages of birth, growth, harvest and storage. Life is just like the change of four seasons of a year. When it is not time for action, one should bury himself in work; when it is time for getting oneself prepared, one should not rush to stand out; when an accidental misfortune comes, it means a greater harvest ahead. When one has such realization and reaches such high realm, it is quite easy for him to keep calm in heart.

**Second, Refrain from Covetousness.** The covetousness of human means the desires for having the things beyond his capability or having the things he does not deserve to have. It stems from the various desires to be satisfied all the time, including the material desires and spiritual desires. The extent of desires satisfaction has become an important happiness index of a man, the higher the desires are satisfied, the better the life will be. In order to satisfy the endless human desires and for better life, man is easy to become covetous and will covet the things beyond his capability or he does not deserve to have. Driven by such covetousness, man will seek more money or power for satisfying the human desires as much as possible or having the things he wishes to have, he will no longer remain a peaceful mind and keep calm. He will rack his mind, feel anxious and will be overworked physically and spiritually, the normal and smooth working of human organs is damaged, seriously over drafting and impairing his heath in a silent way. Through years of accumulation, the various diseases will come to him. So, the covetousness brings about the calamity rather than good health and happiness.

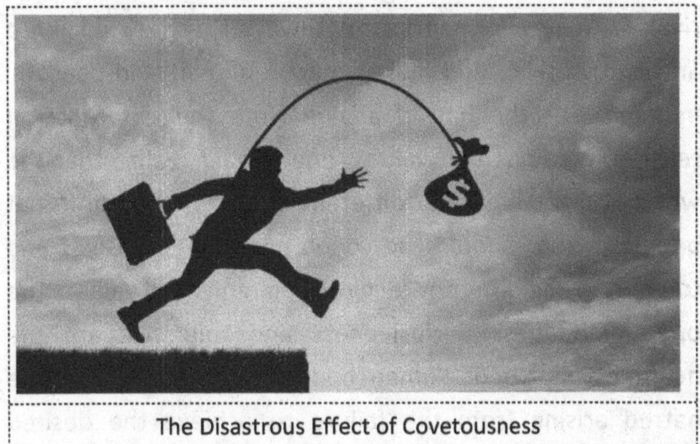

The Disastrous Effect of Covetousness

The Traditional Chinese Medicine (TCM) emphasizes the prevention of diseases rather than curing the diseases. The key to the prevention of disease is to balance the human body and keep the stable mental status, thus avoiding the extreme disastrous effect. To balance the human body and keep the stable mental status, one must curb the excessive human desires, refrain from covetousness and adapt himself to circumstances.

**Third, Refrain from Hatred.** The hatred generally arises from the conflict of interest, competition and struggles, the difference in religion, opinions and values and failure to achieve the desired things, etc. The hatred arising from the conflict of interest, competitions and struggles is primary. The hatred makes man impulsive and impairs the balance of human body, just like the covetousness, causing the mental problems and diseases after long time accumulation. For the hatred arising from the conflict of interest, competitions and struggles, one should devote himself to improving his qualities and capabilities, rather than bear in mind the hatred all the time, in an endeavor to bring him into a better position to compete with the



*Regimen of Good Health and Longevity*

rivals. The success and victory always stay with diligence and hardworking and makes man confident and peaceful in mind. For the hatred arising from the difference in religion, opinions and values, one should realize that the world is diversified and different cultures make different peoples, and should be open-minded, inclusive and tolerant to the different religions, opinions and values. The open-mindedness, inclusiveness and tolerance are the healthiest status of human body and mentality. For the hatred arising from the failure to achieve the desired things, one should reflect on whether the desired things are beyond his capability or he does not deserve to have them. If so, he should no longer seek to have them, otherwise the pain and annoyance will stay with him all the time, causing mental problem and impairing his health; if the desired things are within his capability or should belong to him, he should review and analyze the causes of such failure. In a word, the hatred could do nothing but brings about the affliction and impairs the health.

To achieve good health and longevity, one must cultivate his mentality. Cultivating Mentality is more important than hardworking and struggle for success, it is aimed at making a powerful and calm heart that is not disturbed by outside changes and regards the impermanence as permanence (regards the changes as permanence). A powerful and calm heart is the most crucial capability of a man.

The magic code of Cultivating Mentality is very simple: Calming Mind. It means the continuous improvement of the ability to integrate with the natural to the extent of unity between heaven and man in the end, just like the Taoist Meditation, making the brain and whole cells in a high calm state with nothing in the mind. At this time, the



*Regimen of Good Health and Longevity*

brain is just like superconductor, human experiences the law of things moving in circles and learned the way of nature in an extreme calm mind and in combination with all things. Calming Mind in true sense means that the mood and mentality are immune from the ups and downs and remain stable without complaints, delusion, obsession, wrath, anxiety and terror. Under such condition, the Qi and flood flow smoothly, the human body is naturally free of health problem.

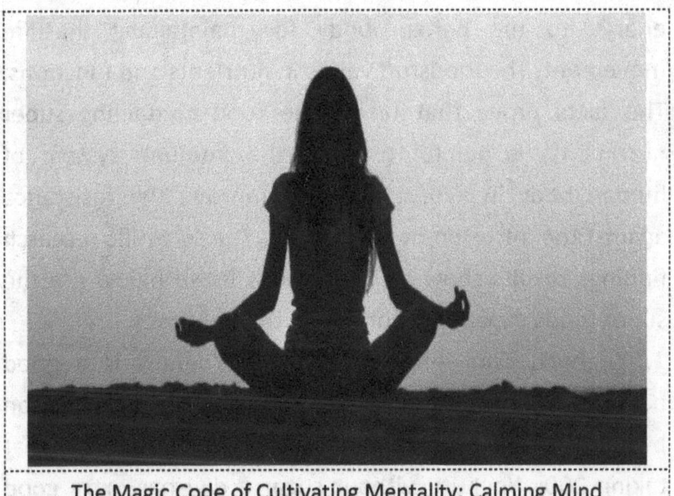

The Magic Code of Cultivating Mentality: Calming Mind

The covetousness, hatred and discomposure are the most fatal enemy to the health of human body. Cultivating Mentality keeps the diseases and viruses away. It has nothing to do with personal achievement, wealth and technology and it is dependent on one's consciousness. Cultivating Mentality more than brings about the good health of human body, more importantly, it opens the innate wisdom and capability of human being.

# Chapter II   Proper Food Taking

Besides the mentality, the health of human body is closely associated with the food taking. The food plays a vital role in promoting and enhancing the health of human body. The primary purpose of food taking is to supplement the energy to the human body for maintaining the life movement. The foodstuff varies in nutrients and functions. The facts prove that taking the food containing super nutriments is helpful to keep the immune system of human body in a best state to improve the resistance against the intrusion by the viruses. The scientific research findings results show that the foods listed below are the super foods capable of enhancing the immunity.

**1. Yoghurt.** The "probiotic" in the Yoghurt is a good bacteria protecting the intestinal tract from the intrusion by Pathogenic Bacteria. A scientific research finds out that taking 200g Yoghurt without sugar a day has extra good effect in enhancing the immunity.

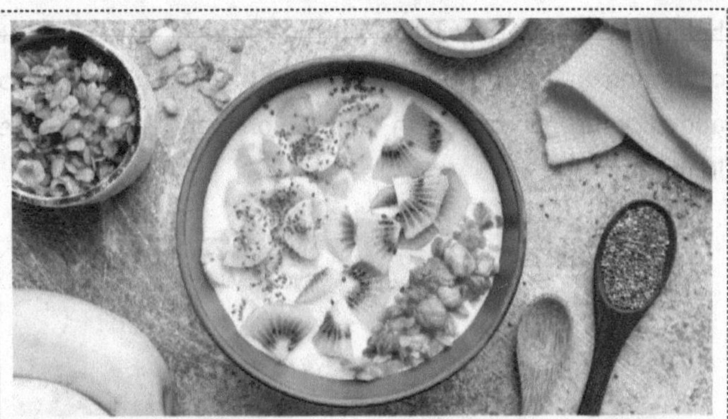

The "probiotic" in the Yoghurt is a good bacteria protecting the intestinal tract from the intrusion by Pathogenic Bacteria

**2. Oats and Barley.**  A scientific research indicates that the oats, barley and other grains contain β—Dextran with high ORAC (Oxygen Radical Absorbance Capacity) that can effectively prevent the influenza and herpes, improve the immunity and accelerate the wound healing, and may promote the better role of antibiotics.

**3. Shellfish.**  The shellfish includes prawn, crab, oyster and clam, etc., it has a rich content of "Selenium".  The protein is one of the important nutrients preserving the immunity, it is also the main constituent of white cell and antibody. When the intake of protein is not adequate, the sufficient white cell and anti-body cannot be produced, leading to the decline of immunity. The "Selenium" contained in the shellfish can stimulate the generation of immune globulin and antibody.

**4. Garlic.**  The research and tests show that eating the garlic can effectively reduce the chance of catching a cold by two thirds.

**5. Chicken soup.**  The chicken soup has anti-inflammatory effects, can alleviate the pain of throat and promote the health of respiratory tract. Furthermore, it can prevent colds and make the bronchus smooth. The chicken soup added with garlic, radish and onion can enhance the immunity.

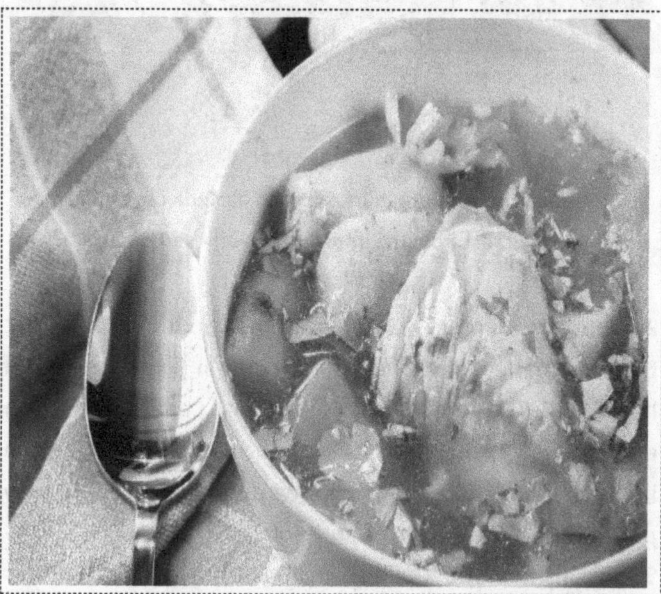

The chicken soup has anti-inflammatory effects, can alleviate the pain of throat and promote the health of respiratory tract.

**6. Tea.** The research shows that the tea has a rich content of amino acid that can improve the immunity. In addition to improving the immunity, drinking tea has great benefits to the health of human body, it can: (1) maintain the normal acid-base balance of blood. The tea contains the alkaloid, including caffeine, theophylline, theobromine and zanthine, etc, it is a good alkaline beverage. The tea can be absorbed and oxidized quickly in the human body, producing the alkaline metabolite of high concentration, thereby the acidic metabolite in the blood is neutralized



*Regimen of Good Health and Longevity*

promptly; (2) delay and prevent the formation of membrane lipid plaque in the blood vessels, thus preventing the arteriosclerosis, hypertension and cerebral thrombosis; (3) can inhibit the malignant tumor and obviously contain the growth of cancer cell; (4) stimulate the spirit, enhance the thinking and memory; (5) dissipate fatigue and promote the metabolism and maintain the normal functioning of heart, blood vessels and stomach intestine, etc.; (6) prevent the dental caries with good effect. A survey indicates that drinking tea can reduce the dental caries of children by 60%; (7) supplement the microelements beneficial to human body; (7) curb the cell aging and prolong life span. The anti-aging effect of tea is more than 18 times better than Vitamin E in this respect; (8) excite the central nervous system and enhance the athleticism; (9) reduce the weight and beautify the skin. Drinking tea ensures the adequate water intake to human body, thereby preserving the elasticity of skin, and metabolizes the toxins existing in the human body, which is beneficial to the skin care. Furthermore, tea has diuretic effect that can take more toxins out of human body, thereby promoting the health of skin, and it has high contents of Vitamin C and chlorophyll with antioxidant effects that can delay the skin aging to some extent; (10) prevent senile cataract; (11) prevent the stomatitis, Pharyngitis, enteritis and diarrhea, etc. incidental in summer as the tannic acid contained in the tea can kill various bacteria; (12) protect the Hematopoiesis of human body. The tea contains anti-radiation substances, which can resist the radiation by electronic products to human body and protect the eyesight; (13) prevent heatstroke and lower temperature. The fact shows that nine minutes later after drinking hot tea, the skin temperature will drop by 1-2 ℃, while cold drinks have no such effect; (14) promote a peaceful mentality. Drinking tea is a slow, quiet and elegant activity, it needs a slow rhythm to carefully taste the fragrance of tea. When the rhythm slows down, the mentality will gradually enter into a quiet and peaceful state, the spiritual pressure and psychosomatic stress will mitigate and be released, thus balancing the human body and preserving the health. So, drinking tea is a regimen with very good effect. In a word, tea is a food of great benefit to health of human body.

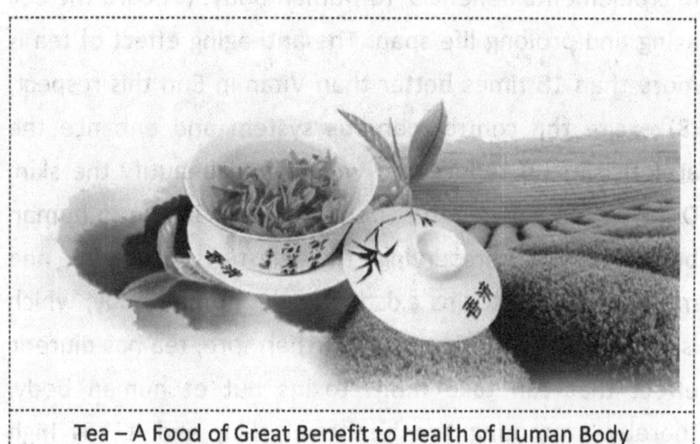

Tea – A Food of Great Benefit to Health of Human Body

**7. Beef.**   The great benefit of the beef is that it has a rich content of various rich minerals constituting the primary sources of immunity of human body, such as magnesium, iron and zinc. The beef has a rich content of protein, its amino acid composition is more close to meet the needs of human body than pork and can enhance the disease resistance. With regard to enhancing immunity, the best value of the beef is that it contains a mineral substance called "Zinc". The Zinc is an antioxidant that is helpful to synthesize the protein and promotes the growth of muscle. Same as glutamate and Vitamin B6, the main function of the Zinc is to enhance the immune system. The Zinc is very important to the development of white cell and it can identify and destroy the outside cells and viruses intruding the human body.

**8. Fresh Fruits and Vegetables.** Skin is a part of immune system and it is the forefront fortress resisting the bacteria, viruses and other unwanted substances. So, it is very important to keep the skin healthy and strong for protecting the health of human body. To this end, the skin needs the Vitamin A, which plays a significant part in generating the connective tissue and is vital to the composition of skin. The best way of supplying Vitamin A to the skin is to eat the food containing $\beta$—carotene, such as Sweet Potatoes, Carrots, Pumpkins and Hami melon, etc. The fresh fruits and vegetables are low in fat, Caloricity and cholesterol, the main nutrients include Vitamin A, Vitamin C, minerals and fibers, etc. Particularly, the orange and dark fruits and vegetables are very beneficial to the health of human body. The fruit juice is not as good as fruits in nutrition, because the pomace, which has rich contents of insoluble dietary fiber and minerals, including potassium and calcium, etc., is discarded when the fruits are crushed and pressed to extract juice, only the sugar and caloricity remain in the juice, the nutrition of fruits is lowered significantly. As more raw materials are consumed in crushing and pressing the fruits, the sugar contained in a cup of juice is likely to be the combination of sugars of several fruits. So, the fruit juice usually has excess sugar content.

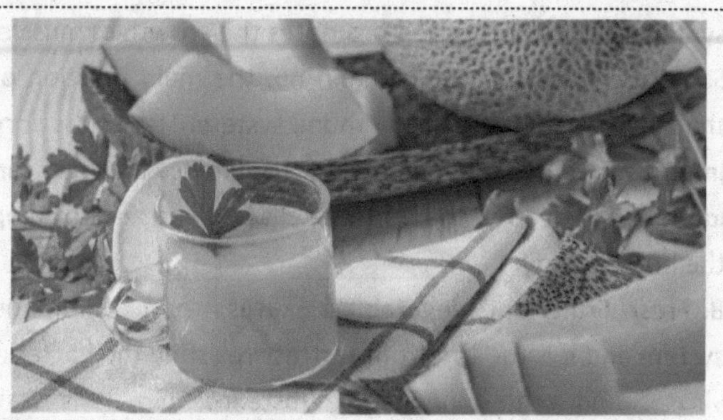

The best way of supplying Vitamin A to the skin is to eat the food containing β—carotene, such as Sweet Potatoes, Carrots, Pumpkins and Hami melon, etc.

**9. Mushroom.** The mushroom is rich in nutrition: the protein content in the mushroom exceeds 30%, much higher than generic vegetables and fruits. It has rich contents of various vitamins and minerals, for instance, calcium and iron. Specifically speaking, the nutrients and minerals contained in the mushroom include protein, fat, saccharide, crude fiber, sodium, potassium, calcium, phosphorus, iron, copper, zinc, manganese, fluorine, polysaccharide, folic acid, nicotinic acid, carotene, Vitamin B1.B2.B6.C,E,K, biotin and various amino acids, such as lactamine and glutamic acid, etc. The most important is that the mushroom contains 8 kinds of amino acids that cannot be synthesized by human body itself and are indispensible to human body.

The fat contains more linoleic acid and less oleic acid. In addition, the mushroom has a rich content of lysine, which is an amino acid necessary to human body, can heighten human body, enhance the disease resistance, increase the Hemoglobin and improve the intelligence. Besides, the mushroom contains interferon inducer capable of inducing the interferon, so, it has quite good therapeutic effect in curing the vesicular stomatitis virus and Encephalitis Viruses, etc. The fresh mushroom extract tablet can cure the persistent hepatitis or chronic hepatitis. The mushroom has the function of lowering the Blood Cholesterol Level, the poptompin and tyrosinase (TYR) contained in the mushroom can lower the blood pressure with obvious effect. Therefore, mushroom is the ideal health-care food to the patients of hypertension and cardiovascular.

The mushroom enjoys very high food therapy values: (1) Enhance the immunity of the organism. After the mushroom is shone by the sunlight, the special substances contained in it are converted into Vitamin D, which is helpful to improve the disease resistance after Vitamin D is absorbed by the human body. Furthermore, the mushroom can stimulate the human body to produce more interferons to kill the viruses in the human body; (2) Ease pain and abirritate. A Brazilian research institute extracted a substance Act—2 from the mushroom, the substance has the effects of easing pain and abirritation and replace the morphine; (3) Relieve cough and reduce sputum. The extracting solution of mushroom, which is used in the experiment on animal, shows that it can relieve cough and reduce sputum; (4) Anti-Cancer. The Japanese research fellows extracted from the mushroom a polysaccharide anti-cancer substance called "PS-K". It is a super-strong anti-cancer substance with a molecular weight of 288 and is 1000 times better than the anti-cancer substances in the green tea in effect. Furthermore, the mushroom contains a toxoprotein that can effectively



*Regimen of Good Health and Longevity*

prevent the protein synthesis of cancer cell; (5) Relaxing the bowels and Detoxifying. The crude fiber, semi-crude fiber and lignin contained in the mushroom and hard to digest in human body can preserve the water in the bowels and absorb the remaining cholesterol and sugar and discharge them out of human body, it is very beneficial to prevent the obstipation, intestinal cancer, arteriosclerosis and diabetes, etc.; (6) Losing Weight. The mushroom has rich contents of nutrition facts, including inorganic substances, vitamins and proteins, etc., they are very low in caloricity. In addition, the mushroom has a very high content of plant cellulose that can prevent constipation and lower the cholesterol level in the blood. The Vitamin C contained in the mushroom is far higher than generic fruits and can promote the metabolism of human body. Besides, the mushroom has very high medical values: the ethanol extract of it can lower the blood sugar, its culture solution has inhibiting effect on the Staphylococcus aureus (S. aureus), Salmonella typhi (S. typhi) and Escherichia coli (E. coli); the mushroom can be used as medicine for curing the weakness of the spleen and the stomach, lack of appetite, fatigue, or hypogalactia of women, cough and adverse rising of visceral energy (adverse flow of Qi). In modern time, the mushroom can also be used as a medicine for curing the infectious hepatitis and leukopenia because it can improve the production and activity of white cell. When the human body is infected with diseases or viruses, the mushroom becomes more resistant and aggressive the disease and viruses. It is a good thing to human body.

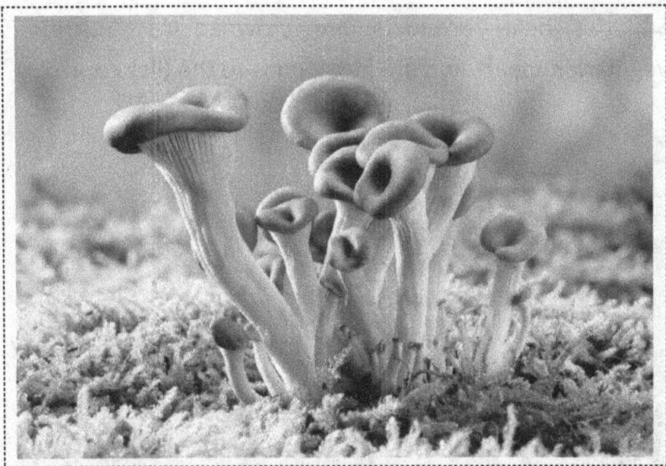

People around the world eat the mushroom to
construct the healthy immune system

Besides, the homonemeae food (including fungus food and seaweed food) has a rich content of polysaccharides that have the effects of anti-cancer and stimulating the immunity and are helpful to protect the cardiovascular of middle-aged and old people.

**10. Oily Fish.** Just like salmon, mackerel and herring, the oily fish has a rich content of Omega－3 fatty acid capable of reducing the inflammation and protecting the lungs or respiratory tract from infection. The result of a research on animals indicates that such nutriment is helpful to resist various flus.

**11. Bean Products.** The bean products have very high contents of protein and Calcium, good satiety and are very low in fat content. Furthermore, the bean products are low in energy conversion efficiency and high in energy consumption. To digest the protein in the bean products, the human body needs to consume the double energy than to consume the same-weight fat and carbohydrate.

21

So, the bean products are crowned as "nutritious vegetarian meat" and are ideal foods to the diet control.

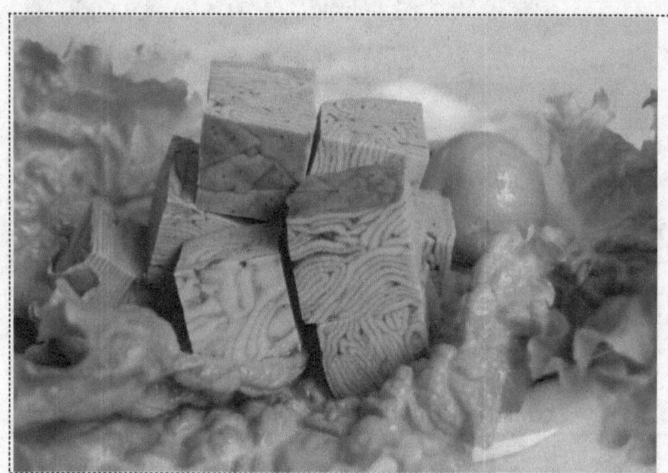

The bean products have very high contents of protein and Calcium, good satiety and are very low in fat content

**12. Propolis.** As a traditional and natural medicine, the Propolis has a history of application more than 2000 years in Europe. Owing to the rich contents of flavone and phenolic acids, the Propolis enjoys very good antioxidant activity and biologic activity. The active ingredients in the Propolis can regulate with good effect the immune system of human body and help to maintain the dynamic balance and relative stability of immune system. The modern research indicates that the rich and unique bioactive substances contained in the Propolis enable the Propolis to have the multiple functions of anti-bacterial, anti-inflammation, relieving itching, antioxidation, enhancing immunity, lowering the blood sugar and blood lipid, and antitumor, etc. The Propolis has extensive and high medical and health values to human body: (1) Regulate the immunity. The Propolis can reinforce the immune system, improve the vitality of immune cell and regulate the adaptive immunity and non-adaptive immunity. The experiments and tests done by the research institutes prove that the Propolis can notably enhance the phagocytosis of macrophage and activity of natural killer cell, increase the antibody production, significantly strengthen the cellular immunity and humoral immunity, make vigorous function adjustment to thymus, spleen and whole immune system, improve the disease resistance, self-curative power or self-healing ability of human body and protect the human body from having diseases or suffering less diseases. The influenza is caused by the virus infection. Whether a person is vulnerable to the influenza, it depends on his immunity. The Propolis can deactivate the influenza virus and enhance the immunity. It is a case in point that those who eat the Propolis products have little chance of having influenza; (2) Purify the blood. The Propolis can improve the cardiac contractility, deepen the breathing, adjust the blood pressure, purify the blood and regulate the blood fat. In 1975, Fang Zhu, a Chinese research fellow and professor, discovered that the Propolis can lower the blood fat. The subsequent massive research and clinical practices prove that the Propolis has evident regulatory effect on the hyperlipemia, hypercholesterolemia and high blood viscosity, can prevent the increase of collagen fiber in the artery vessels and the cholesterol accumulation in the liver, have preventive effect on the atherosclerosis, can effectively clear the deposits in the walls of blood vessel, resist the formation of thrombus, protect the cardiac and cerebral vessels, improve the status of cardiac and cerebral vessels and hematopoiesis. As the Propolis has special effect in purifying the blood, it is called "Blood Vessel Sweeper".

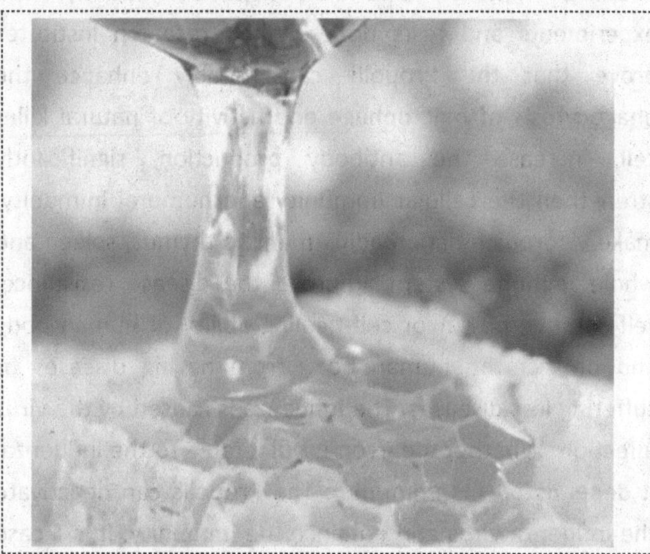

The Propolis Crowned as "Purple Gold" Has Very Good Effect in Anti-Inflammation and Sterilization

Besides, the Propolis and black tea (red tea) have inhibitory effect on the Coronavirus. The polyphenols in the black tea has anti-inflammatory effect. The experiment shows that Catechin can combine with the unicellular bacteria to coagulate and deposit the protein, thereby inhibiting and killing the pathogenic bacteria. The polybase in black tea can absorb, deposit and decompose the heavy metals and alkaloid, protecting modern people from the water and food polluted by industry. The black tea has strong resistance to germs, it can prevent the common cold caused by filterable virus, prevent the tooth decay and food poisoning, lower the blood sugar and hypertension.

# Chapter III     Right Ways of Life

The working of the world where human lives is constrained by the potential underlying logic, just like the Internet products used by people every day are driven by various programs, behind these programs are the initial assumptions and operating logics set by the programmers. The logics that govern the working of the world form an ecosystem. The essence of ecosystem is interconnection, interaction and mutual constraint of the elements existing in the ecology.

In broad sense, Universe is an ecosystem. As a species being on the Earth, human is a small microecology. A large number of microorganisms exist in human body and work with various tissues and organs to drive the movement of human life. They determine the immunity of human body and form a community. When human body gets ill or has problem, it indicates that microorganisms in the human body have problem. The health of human body depends on whether the microorganisms in human body exist in harmony, that is, the health of microorganisms is the health of human body.

To maintain the health of microorganisms in the human body, the key is to keep the balance of human body. Besides cultivating the calm mentality and taking the foods right for enhancing the immunity, the right ways of life is another necessary and important contributor to good health and longevity.

To keep the balance of human body and follow the right ways of life, the things below should be done:

**1. Being Abstemious in Eating and Drinking.** The spleen and stomach are the source of acquired constitution and the source of Qi and blood formation. The balanced and regular dietary habit serve best the care and protection of spleen and stomach, can strengthen the body and enhance the immunity.

The best time for having meals:

Breakfast: 7~9 hours, the food taken can be digest and utilized best;

Lunch: 11~13 hours, the food taken is supplied to the heart after it is converted into energy, it can enhance the vitality of the heart and supply the Qi and blood to the whole body;

Supper: 17~19 hours, the food taken is supplied to the kidney to promote the sleeping and repair the human body.

The principles of taking meals: the breakfast should be replete; the lunch should be good and nutritious; the supper should be less. The contents of meals: the breakfast should be the starchy foods plus meat, egg and dairy; the lunch should be the high-protein foods plus starchy foods, vegetables and fruits; the supper should be the vegetables, fruits and soup. In addition, one should develop the habit of drinking tea, should not eat the fried, smoked, greasy food and roast food as much as possible, refrain from smoking and drinking alcohol, and eating the wild animals.

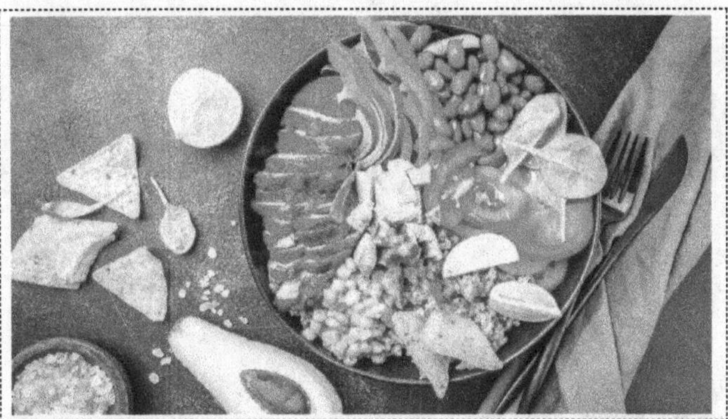

The balanced and regular dietary habit serve best the care and protection of spleen and stomach, can strengthen the body and enhance the immunity.

**2. Having a Light Diet.** The long-lived elders adhere to the principle of having a light diet, namely eat more vegetarian food and less meat dishes. Eating too much meat and fatty food are hard to digest and heavily burden the intestines and stomach. The daily diet should be light dishes and be combined with the vegetables, fruits, coarse grain, meat, eggs and dairy to ensure the overall intake of nutrients.

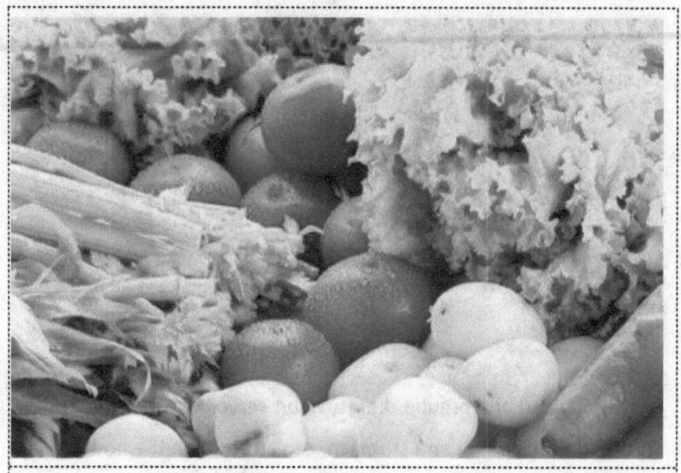
The Light Diet Beneficial to Longevity

It is taken for granted that heath products can promote the health or is beneficial to the health at least. It is a misconception. As a matter of fact, the heath products are the compressed drugs in essence. Eating excessive heath products will cause extreme heavy burden on the intestines, stomach and consume some nutrients and even give rise to some diseases. More vegetables and fruits are recommended in the daily diet for the elderly.

Food is primary to people. The cereals, vegetables, meat, fish and cheese are all the food nourishing human body and supporting the subsistence of people. There is such ancient saying: Meat eaters are vulgar, vegetarians are wise and can live one hundred years. Being satiate all day and remaining idle do harm to human body, not being satiate and remaining in constant light labor are beneficial to human body.

**3. Alternating Work with Rest.** An exercise regimen does not mean that one shall go to Gym Room. There are many ways of exercise regimen. According to the "Huang Di

Canon of Internal Medicine (Huang Di Nei Jing)", the simple and effective way of an exercise regimen is "Working without Fatigue", namely do not fatigue your body in working. Constant light labor keeps the diseases away. Life lies in movement. So, human body should be in motion to promote the circulation of Qi and blood, provided that the motion shall not be excessive or burst the limit, otherwise the internal organs will be hurt, leading to early death. On the other hand, being satiate yet remaining idle all day blocks the smooth circulation of Qi and blood, leading to early aging. Before retirement, working is the primary physical motion of human body. When such physical motion is excessive, it is the overworking, the human body will be "overtired". Following the natural law, man should go to work at sunrise and rest at sunset for good health and longevity. When one feels tired, he should have a rest or dissipate the fatigue in another way. If human body is compared to be a bearing, the rest is the lubricating oil. Overtiring means working without adding lubricating oil. Those long-lived elderly are the persons keeping themselves occupied, or remaining in constant labor without fatigue or overworking, because they do the different things without stubbornness and greed, they do the things within their capabilities and with pleasure. As a matter of fact, they are following the regimen of "Working without Fatigue" and "Constant light labor keeps diseases away".

**4. Leading a Regular Life.**   Human body is a microcosm and is same as the macrocosm in many aspects. The working and rest time of human body is regular. The people in modern time break the normal working and rest time of human body, causing many weird diseases that cannot be identified by hospitals and scientists. Generally speaking, human should fall asleep before 11 hours p.m., and awake after 5 hours a.m. next morning. It is the best rest time for human body because the period from 11 hours p.m. to 5 hours a.m. next morning is the working and recovery time of vital organs of human body, they should not be disturbed, otherwise, the working efficiency of the organs will decline, the blood will not be purified, the organs cannot be repaired, gradually, the human body is prone to aging more quickly and ailing.

# Chapter IV    Foot Bathing ---Soaking Feet

## Section 1    Introduction of Foot Bathing and Its Benefits

### 1. Effects and Benefits of Foot Bathing

The feet of human body is just like the roots of a tree. Foot bathing means soaking feet to warm the whole body and invigorate the internal organs, it is one of the foot therapies of Traditional Chinese Medicine (TCM) and is also a common external therapy. Foot bathing is a means of health care and preservation and is crucial to good health and longevity. It can clear the blood wastes of human body and lesion sediments, dissipate the fatigue and dispel cold, promote sleeping, accelerate blood circulation, stimulate acupuncture points and promote the metabolism. In addition, foot bathing can enhance the immunity of human to resist various diseases. If the hot water is mixed with some traditional Chinese drugs, foot bathing may cure some diseases. For those who get cold feet and hands, foot bathing is a very effective therapy. Foot bathing with hot water is a simple and low-cost family health care option.

Furthermore, foot bathing has very good auxiliary effect in curing many diseases. The sayings "the rich eat restoratives and the poor soak their feet" and "Foot bathing with TCM is better than eating invigorator" are the cases in point. The application of foot bathing with TCM to curing the diseases is wide, which includes the systemic diseases like rheumatism, stomach and spleens diseases,


*Regimen of Good Health and Longevity*

insomnia, arthritis, headache and common cold, and serious illness, such as paraplegia, traumatic brain injury, stroke, Lumbar disc herniation, nephropathy (kidney disease), diabetes, and rehabilitation after serious illness, etc. Foot bathing with hot water can adjust the functions of internal organs and improve the physique. For healthy people, foot bathing with fresh water or salt water or vinegar water is enough for health preservation, it is a simple and low-cost regimen.

The foot is also called the "Second Heart" of human body and it is regarded as the "Root of Vital Essence and Energy (Genuine Energy)". The scientific research proves that the feet are the hub of meridians and collaterals and distributed with more than 60 acupoints, and have the reflection zones that correspond to the internal organs of human body and channel distribution. When the feet are soaked in hot water, these reflection zones are stimulated, thus promoting the blood circulation, regulating the endocrine system, enhancing the functions of human organs and preventing the diseases. Meanwhile, the hot water stimulation accelerates the microcirculation of the feet and opens the trichopore, making more blood flow to the peripheral vessel of lower extremity and reducing the blood flowing to the brain, thereby, the sense of drowsiness comes up. On the other hand, as numerous nerve endings on the sole of feet are closely connected with the brain, the hot water stimulation on these nerve endings produces the inhibitory effect on cerebral cortex, making the brain relaxed and comfortable, thus promoting and deepening the sleeping. Besides, foot bathing aided with traditional Chinese medicines can assist the treatment of many diseases and dissipate the cold in the human body.

Foot bathing is applicable around the year and has different effects in four seasons. Generally speaking, foot bathing in spring can enhance the Yang Qi (Positive Energy) of human body to prevent the prolapse of internal organs. Yang Qi is a combination of innate Qi inherited from parent, the Qi from respiration and the Qi converted from the vital essences of food. Yang Qi is the source power of metabolism and physical functions of human body and it is the determinant of production, growth, development, aging and death of human body. It can warm and nourish the whole body tissues and preserve the functions of internal organs. The normal existence and activities of human body, including the mood fluctuations, adapting to temperature change and repairing the wounds, etc., all consume the Yang Qi. When the Yang Qi is weak, the physical activities of human body will decrease and decline. The diseases, such as prolapse of uterus and gastroptosis, etc., are caused by the decline of Yang Qi. Foot bathing in spring has therapeutic effect on such diseases; Foot bathing in summer can dispel dampness and eliminate heat, prevent the common cold, refresh vitality, stimulate appetite, promote sleeping and enhance the functions of internal organs. Foot bathing in autumn can moisten the lungs and intestines. Foot bathing in winter can nourish and invigorate heart and kidney.

**2. Necessary Conditions of Foot Bathing.** First, get ready for the right foot bathing barrel. A right foot bathing barrel is important for having good effect. The foot bathing barrel shall be safe, free of harm and have good thermal insulation. The wooden barrel with smart temperature regulator is preferred, the height of foot bathing barrel shall be over 20 centimeters so that the ankle joint can be immersed; Second, regulate the temperature of foot bathing water to 38~43℃, not exceeding 45℃ at most, the proper foot bathing time is 15~30 minutes; Third, confirm the foot bathing effect. When the back moistens or the light sweat comes out of forehead, it indicates that the meridians and collaterals of human body are connected up and the effect of foot bathing is realized. The profuse sweat is prohibited in foot bathing as it will hurt the heart.

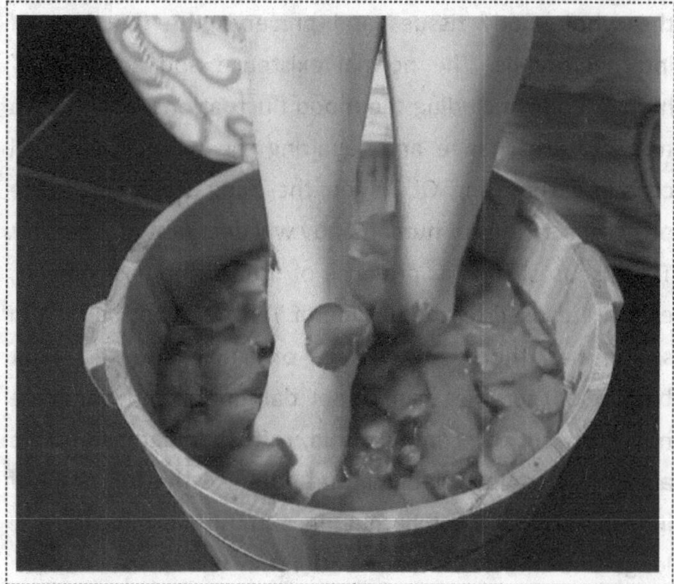

Foot bathing ---A Simple and Low-Cost Family Health Care Option

# Section 2    TCM Prescriptions for Foot Bathing

Foot bathing in pure hot water is a very good health-care way and can produce the above-mentioned effects and benefits. If the hot water is mixed with some Traditional Chinese Medicine (TCM) prescriptions, foot bathing is a green and effective external therapy for some diseases. The proved common TCM prescriptions for foot bathing are recommended as follows:

**1. Foot Bathing with Artemisia Argyi.** It is a time-honored and most common foot bathing therapy. The method is very simple: Put 50~100g Artemisia Argyi into water (the amount of water is not fixed) and boil the water up. Soak the feet in the water when the temperature of the water remains at 40~50℃ and soak the feet in the water for 15 ~30 minutes, do it once a week. Foot bathing with Artemisia Argyi can dispel asthenic fire and cold fire with good effect, and can cure the oral ulcer, swelling and pain in throat, periodontitis, gingivitis and tympanitis, etc. To eliminate the discomfort on the head, face and throat, which arise from the asthenic fire and cold fire, it needs to have foot bathing for consecutive 2-3 days before going to bed. Besides, Foot Bathing with Artemisia Argyi can prevent cold, alleviate the headache and improve the resistance of human body against diseases. It had better drink a bowl of syrup after foot bathing with Artemisia Argyi.

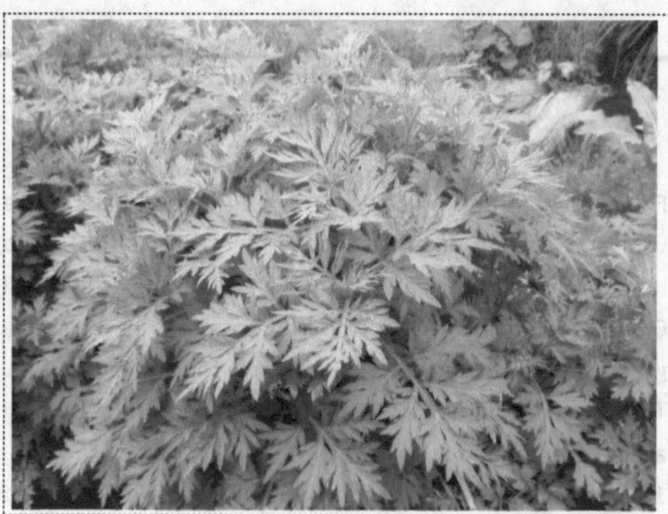

Artemisia Argyi – An Important and Widely-Used Chinese Herbal
Medicine with High Medical Values

Besides the volatile oil as its main content, Artemisia Argyi contains tannins, flavone, alcohol, polysaccharide, microelements and other organic components. In terms of Pharmacological Actions, the modern experiments and research prove that the Artemisia Argyi has the effects of anti-bacteria, anti-virus, relieving asthma, relieving cough, dispelling phlegm, ananaphylaxis, hemostasis and anti-coagulation, sedation, protecting livers and promoting choleresis, and enhance the immunity, etc.; in regard of clinical practice, Artemisia Argyi is widely applied in curing the gynecological diseases, such as uterine bleeding and dysmenorrhea, etc., and respiratory diseases, such as bronchitis, tuberculosis and common cold, etc.

The traditional theory of drug property holds that Artemisia Argyi has the medical effects of recuperating Qi (vital energy) and blood, reinvigorate vitality, dispel cold and damp, warming the channels, hemostasis and miscarriage prevention, etc. Furthermore, Artemisia Argyi is used to make the diets of "Artemisia Argyi Tea", "Artemisia Argyi Soup", "Artemisia Argyi Porridge", etc., to improve the resistance of human body against diseases.

The pharmacological research of modern medicine indicates that Artemisia Argyi is a broad-spectrum antibacterial and anti-virus medicine, it can inhibit and kill many viruses and bacteria, and has protective and therapeutic effects on the respiratory diseases.

Artemisia Argyi is widely used as medicine in China for curing the diseases since the ancient time. The modern technology opens broader prospect for wide application of Artemisia Argyi. Now a series of Artemisia Argyi products, such as Artemisia Argyi toothpaste and bath preparation, Artemisia Argyi oil essence, pillow and mosquito-repellent incense, etc., are developed. Now a cigarette with Artemisia Argyi as main raw material is being developed, it has no content of nicotine and can be used as substitute of cigarette.

Artemisia Argyi is mainly distributed in East Asia, it is an adaptable plant that grows on roadside and grassland. As a Chinese herbal medicine that can be obtained locally and widely, Artemisia Argyi is used a primary medicine for preventing the pandemic since the ancient time, Fumigating Artemisia Argyi is a simple and easy method of preventing the pandemic.

There are some proved recipes for foot bathing with Artemisia Argyi plus some materials: (1) Artemisia Argyi added with ginger can cure the flu caused by wind and cold, arthropathy, Rheumatoid Arthritis, coughing, bronchitis, pulmonary emphysema and asthma; (2) Artemisia Argyi added with Safflower (red flower) can improve varicosity, terminal neuritis, poor blood circulation, numbness in hands and feet or blood stasis; (3) Artemisia Argyi added with salt can cure the endogenous heat of upper thorax (heart and lungs), red eyes, toothache, throat sore, vexation and impatience, asthenia fire in upper thorax and cold in abdomen, legs and feet swelling; (4) Artemisia Argyi added with 20 wild peppers can cure the foot sweat, foot odor, beriber and eczema.

**2. Foot Bathing with Eaglewood Powder.** It can improve the blood circulation, alleviate fatigue, dispel cold, promote metabolism, dredge meridians and collaterals, regulate Qi and invigorate blood.

**3. Foot Bathing Prescription for Removing Foot Order.** There are four prescriptions: (1) take a half daikon, cut it into thin pieces, boil them in pot for 3 minutes with big fire, then cook them with mild fire for 5 minutes, then pour the cooled water into bathing barrel and soak the feet in it, do it several times; (2) grind 1~2 pieces of Oxytetracycline into fine powder, spread the fine powder between the toes, soak the feet in hot water, do it without a break, the foot order will be removed half a month later; (3) Put appropriate amount of salt and several pieces of ginger into hot water, soak the feet into hot water and scrub the feet for several minutes, the foot order will be removed and the fatigue is dissipated; (4) Soak the feet in the vinegar water. Put 100~150g rice vinegar or mature vinegar into hot water, then soak the feet in the hot water for 15~20 minutes. The foot bathing with vinegar can: (i) remove the foot order, kill the bacteria and cure the beriber to some extent; (ii) relieve fatigue; (iii) eliminate rheumatism (wind-damp) and improve the symptom of fearing cold and chill; (iv) moisturize the skin, soften the horniness and enhance skin elasticity; (v) cure the sleep disorder; (vi) enhance blood circulation, clear the blood wastes and lesion dregs and cure some chronic ailments after the vinegar penetrates into the surface skin of feet.

**4. Foot Bathing Prescription for Insomnia (Sleeplessness ).** Ingredient: 20g Fructus Schisandrae (Schisandra Chinensis, fruit of Chinese Magnoliavine), 20g Rhizoma Cyperi (Cyperus Rotundus), 30g Tuber Fleeceflower Stem, 30g Turmeric, 30g Ligusticum Wallichii (Szechuan Lovage Rhizome) and 30g Rhizoma Acori Tatarinowii (Acorus Gramineus). Method: Wrap the ingredients with cotton gauze and boil them in water for 50 minutes, then mixed them with the water in the foot bathing barrel. When the water temperature falls to 40°C, soak the feet in the water for 30 minutes, do it once a day and repeat it for 2~3 days.

**5. Foot Bathing Prescription for Dispersing Cold by Warming the Meridians.** Ingredients: 30g old ginger, 30g Stauntonia hexaphylla, 30g Radix Gentianae Macrophyllae, 20g Cinnamomum cassia, 30g Radix Angelicae Pubescentis, 30g Radix Cynanchi Paniculati, 30g Zanthoxylum schinifolium (Pepper) and 15g red flower (flowers carthami) Method: wrap the ingredients with cotton gauze, boil them in water for 50 minutes, then mix them with the water in the foot bathing barrel. When the water temperature falls to 40°C, soak the feet in the water for 30 minutes, the cold will be dispersed and meridians will be warmed.

**6. Foot Bathing Prescription for Improving Sleeping Quality.** Add pebbles to the water in the foot bathing barrel, rub the feet on the pebbles, it can enhance the foot bathing effect, promote the connection of meridians and collaterals, keep the heart in communication with the kidney, disperse and rectify the depressed liver-energy, strengthen the spleen and replenish Qi, calm the heart and tranquilize the mind (relieve mental stress). Rubbing the feet with pebbles while having a foot bathing can produce the effect similar to acupuncture and moxibustion and better improving the sleeping quality. The foot bathing water temperature shall remain at 45°C and the foot bathing shall last 20~30 minutes.

**7. Foot Bathing Prescription for Tinea Pedis, Leg Itch, Sweaty Feet and Stinky Feet.** Ingredients: Cortex Phellodendri Chinensis, Drgon's bones, alums, Flos Sophorae, Galla Chinensis, Turmeric, Clove, Sophora flavescens Ait, Rheum palmatum, fructus kochiae and Sanguisorba officinalis. Effect: clear away heat and toxic materials, destroy parasites and relieve itching.

**8. Foot Bathing Prescription for Middle-Aged and Elderly Lumbocrural Pain.** Ingredients: Saposhnikovia divaricate, East Asian Tree Fern Rhizome, Salvia miltiorrhiza, Radix Astragali and Angelica sinensis. Effect: Tonify liver and kidney, nourish Qi and blood, disperse wind and dampness and connect meridians and collaterals, cure the deficiency of liver-kidney deficiency, insufficiency of vital energy (Qi) and blood and lumbocrural pain of middle-aged and elder people.

**9. Foot Bathing Prescription for Nourishing the Blood and Replenishing Vital Essence of Gynecology.** Ingredients: Salvia miltiorrhiza, parched wild jujube seed, roasted malt, Rice-grain Sprout, Radix Rehmanniae Preparata, Chinese Angelica, dogwood, Radix Polygalae, Schisandra chinensis, Radix Aconiti lateralis Preparata, root of herbaceous peony, fruit of Chinese wolfberry and Semen Cuscutae. Effect:

Nourish the blood and replenishing vital essence, regulate and replenish liver and kidney, applicable to sterility due to deficiency of the blood.

**10. Foot Bathing Prescription for Relieving Qi Stagnancy in Liver and Harmonize the Stomach and Fortify the Spleen.** Ingredients: Angelica sinensis, dried tangerine or orange peel, Green Tangerine Peel, fructus amomi, Red Kojic Rice, clove, Fructus Hordei Germinatus, Fructus Aurantii, Gardenia jasminoides, bark of magnolia, Agastache rugosa and Radix Aucklandiae. Effect: Applicable to Liver depression and qi stagnation, disharmony between spleen and stomach, indigestion and rib-side distention and pain of the elderly.

**11. Foot Bathing Prescription for Relieving Stress and Mitigating Fatigue.** Ingredients: Cinnamon, Acanthopanax senticosus, licorice, Ginseng leaf, Ligusticum wallichii, Polygonum multiflorum, sharpleaf galangal fruit and Semen Cuscutae. Effect: Disperse wind and dampness, nourish liver and kidney and strengthen the bones and muscles, applicable to the lack of sleep and heavy mental pressure after strenuous exercise and long-time working or physical labor, and Chronic fatigue syndrome, such as inattention, fatigued and weak and muscle soreness, lack of appetite, etc.

**12. Foot Bathing Prescription for Nourishing Yin and Strengthening Yang for Stimulating Sexual Desire, Enhancing Potency and Prolonging Life.** Ingredients: Allium tuberosum Rottl. (Chinese leek seed), Morindae Officinalis, Eucommia ulmoides Oliver, Codonopsis pilosula, astragalus membranaceus, Barbary Wolfberry Fruit (fruit of Chinese wolfberry), bull penis, Cistanche deserticola, Prepared Rehmannia Root, Semen Cuscutae (seed of Chinese dodder) and fresh ginger. Effect: warm the kidney and reinforce the vital functions, fortify the sperm and enhance sexuality, applicable to backache, inability of tibia, prospermia and impotence arising from kidney Yang (energy) deficiency.

**13. Foot Bathing Prescription for Chronic Bronchitis.** Ingredients: loguat leaf, root bark of white mulberry, Bulbus Fritillariae Thunbergii, dried tangerine or orange peel, Pinellia ternate, herba houttuyniae, platycodon grandiflorum and perilla fruit. Effect: cure the chronic bronchitis.

**14. Foot Bathing Prescription for Insomnia.** Ingredients: astragalus membranaceus, largehead atractylodes rhizome, dried tangerine or orange peel, Codonopsis pilosula, Angelica sinensis, licorice, rattletop and radix bupleuri. Effect: invigorate spleen-stomach and replenish Qi, relieve Qi Stagnancy in Liver (sooth the liver), cure the insomnia.

**15. Foot Bathing Prescription for Chronic Gastritis.** Ingredients: Agastache rugosa, Herba Eupatorii, Eggshell, Angelica sinensis, dried tangerine or orange peel, Red Yeast Rice, fructus amomi and clove. Effect: Relieving Qi Stagnancy in Liver, regulate stomach-qi and alleviate pain, activate stagnancy and resolve dampness, applicable to chronic   gastritis, and indigestion and stomach distending pain caused by disharmony between spleen and stomach.

**16. Foot Bathing Prescription for Hyperlipidemia.** Ingredients: fruit of Cherokee rose, Cassia Seed, prepared fleece flower root (Polygonum Multiflorum Thunb), raw coix seed, Herba Artemisiae Scopariae, rhizome of oriental water plantain, raw hawthorn, Radix Bupleuri, Turmeric and rhubarb root parched in wine (Jiu Da Huang). Effect: nourish yin to reduce fire, remove stagnation and invigorate pulse-beat, applicable to cure hyperlipidemia.

**17. Foot Bathing Prescription for Hypertension.**
Ingredients: Concha Haliotidis, Apocynum venetum, Herba
Siegesbeckiae, Herba Taxilli, Salvia miltiorrhiza, root of
herbaceous peony, Stephania tetrandra. Effect: Nourish
the liver and kidney, lower blood pressure and calm the
wind, clear away summer-heat and replenish Qi, calm the
liver and subdue Yang (heat or fire), applicable to cure
headaches, anxiety and irritability and waist and knee
pains arising from essential hypertension.

**18. Foot Bathing Prescription for Diabetes.** Ingredients:
Cassia Twig, Prepared Common Monkshood Daughter
Root, Salvia miltiorrhiza, Honeysuckle Stem, raw milkvetch
root, Olibanum and myrrh. Effect: Warm Yang to restore
normal collateral, promote blood circulation to dispel
blood stasis, clear away heat and toxic materials, dispel
wind and dampness, relieve pain and promote granulation,
applicable to cure the Diabetes.

19. Foot Bathing Prescription for Obesity. Ingredients:
Rhizoma Polygonati, Rhizoma Zingiberis, Cinnamomum
cassia, Waxgourd Peel, Polygonum multiflorum and
Fructus Sophorae (sophora fruit). Effect: Induce diuresis to
alleviate edema, clear heat and remove dampness and
lower fat and reduce weight, applicable to cure the simple
obesity, hyperlipidemia and arteriosclerosis.

**20. Foot Bathing Prescription for Rheumatoid Arthritis.**
Ingredients: Lightyellow Sophora Root, Rhizoma
Atractylodis, Zanthoxylum bungeanum (Pricklyash Peel),
Cortex Phellodendri, Saposhnikovia divaricate, Herba
Schizonepetae, Licorice, Angelica sinensis and Tree Peony
Bark. Effect: Expel wind evil and clear away cold, promote
blood circulation to remove meridian obstruction, remove


*Regimen of Good Health and Longevity*

dampness and relieve pain and strengthen the muscles and bones, applicable to cure the rheumatic lumbocrural pain, arthralgia and myalgia caused by wind-cold attack, the swelling and pain after soft tissue injury, and chronic low back pain.

**21. Foot Bathing Prescription for Climacteric Syndrome.** Ingredients: Rhizoma Coptidis, Semen Ziziphi Spinosae, Radix Ophiopogonis, Radix Paeoniae Alba, Radix Cynanchi Atrati, Salvia miltiorrhiza, Drgonsbones (Fossilizid). Effect: nourish the liver and kidney, calm the liver and lower the evil fire, Nourish yin and suppress hyperactive yang, nourish blood and tranquilize mind, applicable to cure the climacteric syndrome.

**22. Foot Bathing Prescription for Magic Ginger Therapy.** Ingredients: dried ginger, Wild Chrysanthemum, Rhizoma Atractylodis, Folium Artemisiae Argyi, Angelica sinensis, Ligusticum wallichii, Flos Caryophyllata (Clove), Cocklour Fruit (Fructus Xanthii) and Herb of Wild Mint (Peppermint). Effect: Dispel the wind and cold, activate the collaterals and invigorate pulse-beat, warm the spleen and stomach to dispel cold, replenish Qi and blood, particularly effective for curing the cool extremities caused by chilblain and impaired blood circulation.

Warnings for Foot Bathing: (i) Not have a foot bathing within half an hour after meal as it will affect the blood supply to stomach and lead to malnutrition; (ii) Not go to sleep right away after foot bathing; (iii) Not read or watch TV or do other thing while having a foot bathing, it had better close your eyes and calm your mind in foot bathing so that the heat can flow downward to warm the kidneys.

**23. Foot Bathing Prescription for Recuperating Dysmenorrhea and Promoting Blood Circulation to**

**Remove Stasis.**     Ingredients: Salvia miltiorrhiza, Red Peony Root, Herba Lycopi, Semen Vaccariae, Angelica sinensis, radix et rhizoma rhei, Radix Achyranthis Bidentatae and Ligusticum wallichii.

**24. Foot Bathing Prescription for Relieving Wind-Damp Pain.** Ingredients:    Old Ginger, Cinnamomum cassia, Radix Achyranthis Bidentatae, Radix Gentianae Macrophyllae, Herba Lycopi, Ramulus Mori, Angelicae Pubescentis Radix, Red Peony Root, Radix Cynanchi Paniculati and Radix Stephaniae Tetrandrae.

**25. Foot Bathing Prescription for Improving Kidney Asthenia.** Ingredients:    Tremolite (Actinolite), Semen Cuscutae, Fructus Foeniculi, Cortex Cinnamomi, rhizome of rehmannia, Common Cnidium Fruit and  Semen Euryales.

**26. Foot Bathing Prescription for Improving Sub-Health Status.**   Ingredients: Radix Codonopsis, Radix Astragali, Poria, Rhizoma Atractylodis Macrocephalae, Ligusticum wallichii, Pericarpium Citri Reticulatae and Grassleaf Sweelflag Rhizome (Drug Sweetflag Rhizome).

### Section 3    Scientific Basis for Foot Bathing Regimen

The foot bathing regimen has scientific basis: First, skin is one of the organs of human body, it has the functions of shielding and absorbing, secretions and excretions, temperature regulation, feeling and breathing. As skin itself can absorb the medicine, it can facilitate the effect of

45

medicine throughout the human body with aid of hot water; second, foot is one of the hubs of meridians through which Qi and blood (vital energy) circulates. Among 12 regular meridians of human body, 3 Yang meridians of foot end at the foot and 3 Yin meridians of the foot starts from the foot. The 66 meridian acupuncture points are distributed at the feet. Foot bathing with TCM can stimulate these acupuncture points, regulate the meridians, promote flow of Qi and blood and adjust the function of internal organs, thus preventing and curing the diseases.

The scientific basis of foot bathing regimen comes from the Four Theories below:

**(1) Holographic Theory.** Biological holographic theory points out that the feet have the reflection zones corresponding to the internal organs of human body. Stimulating these reflection zones in the feet can regulate the physiological functions of internal organs of human body, thus curing the disease and promoting the self-health care. The feet have 62 basic reflection zones and are like a microcosm that watches the health condition of the parts of human body. Stimulating the reflection zones by foot bathing with TCM can enhance the intake of the medicine and accelerate the distribution of the medicine, promote the smooth flow of blood, regulate the functions of tissues and organs, improve the pathologic changes of internal organs, thus strengthening the immunity of human body.

**(2) Meridians Theory.** Foot is one of the hubs of meridians, 3 Yang meridians of foot end at the foot and 3 Yin meridians of the foot starts from the foot. The 66 meridian acupuncture points are distributed at the feet.

46

These acupuncture points are closely connected with internal organs of human body and very sensitive to various stimulations. Foot bathing with TCM can promote flow of Qi and blood and warm the internal organs, thus curing the internal diseases with external therapy.

**(3) Circulation Theory.** The foot is most far away from the heart and receives the blood supply less than other parts of human body. The heat effect and medicine effect of foot bathing drive and promote the blood circulation throughout the human body and excrete the toxins and wastes out of human body through metabolism, the medical ions are transmitted to the whole body with blood circulation through meridians and collaterals, thus curing the diseases and preserving the health.

**(4) Physics Theory.** In foot bathing with TCM, under the co-actions of heat, water pressure, medical ion movement and other physical agents, the feet are stimulated to trigger the self-regulation of human body, promote the human body to produce resistance and strengthen the immunity, thereby inhibiting or reducing the release of bioactive substance, regulating the metabolism of internal organs, preventing and curing the diseases. Meanwhile, under the action of biologic negative ion energy, the nerve cell of pituitary gland, cerebral gland and lymphocyte are activated in full measure, therefore enhancing antibody substance's capability of identifying and killing the pathogenic bacteria and viruses, promoting the excretion of toxins out of human body through excretion organs, including sweat gland and urinary system.

# Chapter V  Conclusion

Human is the product of natural world. The stable and normal working (or good health) of natural world (the Earth) depends on the balance of ecosystem. When the ecosystem loses balance, the natural disasters and plagues will come up. It is the symptom that the natural "gets ill". The Ecosystem imbalance is usually caused by outside or man-made factors, such as overexploitation, pollution, the production and life activities of human being, etc. Human body is a similar to the natural in this respect. The diseases of human is caused by outside factors in most circumstances, including the volatile mood, improper food taking and irregular ways of life and lack of health care knowledge and skills, etc.

Qi (vital energy) and blood are the sources of the vitality of human body and the smooth flow of Qi and blood is the key to the balance of human body. When the Qi (vital energy) and blood are blocked or cannot flow smoothly, the internal organs cannot work normally and properly, human body will lose the balance, the diseases come up. So, to achieve good health and longevity, maintaining the balance of human body is essential. To this end, one must: (i) cultivate his mind to keep a good mood so that the balance of human body is maintained and internal organs are free of injury; (ii) take proper food that can enhance the immunity to resist the diseases and viruses; (iii) follow the right ways of life to orientate the human body to natural rules and outside environment; (iv) have foot bathing on regular basis. Going to a doctor and taking medicine are the outside intervention means for recovering the balance of human body and restoring the normal functions (working) of internal organs.

In a word, to keep the doctors and drugs away and achieve good health and longevity, the regimens are simple: refrain from excessive desires, keep a good mood, maintain the balance of human body, take the proper food, following natural rules and adapt to outside environment and circumstances.

---The End---